Good Midnight, Insomniacs:
Waking up from Depression
and Addiction to Discovery.

Alma Cosgrove, PhD.

Copyright 2021
iUniverse

GOOD MIDNIGHT, INSOMNIACS

To Frank:
DUM SPIRO SPERO!!

I don't know what to write right now,

Yours always,
Alma

September 12, 2012
Valley House

GOOD MIDNIGHT, INSOMNIACS:

Waking up from Depression and Addiction to Discovery

Alma Christova, PhD

iUniverse, Inc.
Bloomington

GOOD MIDNIGHT, INSOMNIACS
WAKING UP FROM DEPRESSION AND ADDICTION TO DISCOVERY

Copyright © 2012 by Alma Christova, PhD.

All rights reserved. No part of this book may be used or reproduced by any means, graphic, electronic, or mechanical, including photocopying, recording, taping or by any information storage retrieval system without the written permission of the publisher except in the case of brief quotations embodied in critical articles and reviews.

iUniverse books may be ordered through booksellers or by contacting:

iUniverse
1663 Liberty Drive
Bloomington, IN 47403
www.iuniverse.com
1-800-Authors (1-800-288-4677)

Because of the dynamic nature of the Internet, any web addresses or links contained in this book may have changed since publication and may no longer be valid. The views expressed in this work are solely those of the author and do not necessarily reflect the views of the publisher, and the publisher hereby disclaims any responsibility for them.

Any people depicted in stock imagery provided by Thinkstock are models, and such images are being used for illustrative purposes only.
Certain stock imagery © Thinkstock.

ISBN: 978-1-4697-7833-4 (sc)
ISBN: 978-1-4697-7834-1 (ebk)

Printed in the United States of America

iUniverse rev. date: 03/20/2012

CONTENTS

1. Author's Warning:... ix
2. Acknowledgements xvii
3. Introduction... xxi
4. My Life Story for Alcoholics Anonymous 1
5. My ACDC Experience: Recovery begins with ACDC, expands with AA, WfS, DRA, SS, Equilibrium etc. 12
6. Planet Papillon and Life after ACDC.............................. 22
7. 'Living on the Hyphen': Curse or Blessing?..................... 28
8. Sober Love 30
9. Eternal Emails 31
10. Conclusion 33
11. References, Resources and Recommendations................ 37
12. Photo Albums 43

To Ahi

In legal terms my son embodies my untouchable prosecutor at times of crime, my all successful defense lawyer when I opted for a trial and my silent witness at sentencing. In spiritual terms, he must have been always my Higher Power but I had no clue until I finally joined Alcoholics Anonymous last July. And Ahi, thank you from the bottom of my heart for diligently executing all these jobs on my behalf PRO BONO.

AUTHOR'S WARNING:

My dear Reader,

Since this is a self-published book, it is—of course—highly disorganized. Let's think of it as a spontaneous collage of information and pictures put together in one single breath and sent to you as a snail letter (or an email, a facebook entry, a skype call) in my attempt to document the beginning of my recovery from addiction and depression. I neurotically hastened to report everything I learned and experienced in the past eight months in order to share the impact of the Day Treatment Program at the Addictions and Concurrent Disorders Centre at Credit Valley Hospital in Mississauga. To tell you the truth, I think that publishing my sunrise pictures alone would be more than enough to inspire even the most depressed insomniac on earth, but since I paid iUniverse, why not let you know more things about me. So as a true insomniac, always in the wee hours of the morning, I started filing journal entries, diligent notes from my program and aftercare, some "eternal emails", positive quotes of the day, references to the tones of books I have read, summaries of the meetings of the self-help groups I joined in the meantime, then more pictures etc. All in the file "AAA: Alcoholic Anonymous Alma". Once I mentioned on Facebook that I joined AA, I immediately got a lot of suggestions what "Triple A" could stand for. I am sure my reader will come up with many more, funnier and optimistic or pessimistic. I would love to hear them from you for my collection. I so much wanted to have an "AAA" tattoo on my right shoulder and a small butterfly on my left shoulder. Never got the time to do it, believe it or not, but kept buying temporary tattoos from the Dollarama and always had them on. My friend AA34—a gentleman with at least 100 real tattoos—keeps making fun of me that I don't have the guts for a real one.

Things continued to happen every single day and my AAA file started piling up considerably. Christmas—my internal deadline—was approaching fast and I found myself having written much more than I planned back in August 2011. I obviously talk a lot and one has to be brutal to shut me up. If I kept describing the daily events it would have taken us to infinity. Gotthold Ephraim Lessing once said: "My dear friend, I am sending you a long letter because I don't have the time to write you a short one". Hahahaaa. It's so true. My next booklet will be much more concise, I promise. This one is rather a reanimation breath of someone who almost died, but then (for SOME reason) was granted a "life-rebirth-type of breath" and had this crucial vital grasp of air and so was enabled to remain alive for the time being. Something like this. I hope you know what I mean because I don't know the term for this type of breath—I am sure I can ask a specialist of course and I will keep you posted. This breath I couldn't refuse—it meant staying alive. Now that "Good Midnight, Insomniacs" is on your screen, I can readily share with you that my next project is a sitcom entitled "SOBER CHAOS" and features my most precious AA characters and I dare to say that it is going to be FUNNY!! And it will supply fame and money. In order to protect her anonymity and to give her some space, I deliberately excluded my one and only best friend and sober sister AA01 from this booklet although she plays an enormous part in my recovery. Our friendship got so intense over the past 8 months that it would be suffocating to even try to include it here. AA01 is the main character of my sitcom and she deserves my full attention (and yours, trust me) in my next project. She is my golden mine and my ticket to Hollywood. Here I need to mention only that AA01's husband (a wonderful man and a great supporter of our sobriety cause) was the first person to learn that

I FINALLY came up with the title of my book after struggling for three months and having bombarded their family with over twenty possible ideas. I called hysterically very early one morning and he was the one who picked up the phone. He said: "Good. Now try to get some sleep please". He sounded happy and relieved. Thank you AA01 and AA01's Hubby—I am so glad you are part of my future.

As for my file "Bulgarian Crime in Ontario" created on a daily basis since I started interpreting in the courts of the province, it will be published 'post mortum' by my son Chris because I don't want to be prosecuted or killed by its heroes. (Hahahaa, Ahi, the password is "Estrogen". Capital "E" if sensitive.)

Anyways, back to business, as I mentioned already, here you will find a selection from my almost four thousand pictures of the sunrise taken from the balcony of my penthouse since the beginning of August 2011. They represent the triumph of hope over despair; the glimpse of future to what seemed a dead end; the optimistic healing over my depression and addiction. In the piece of prose "Yesterday, Today and Tomorrow" which is read at every AA meeting in my area, there is the following line: "Tomorrow's sun will rise either in splendor or behind a mask of clouds—but it will rise. And until it does, we have no stake in tomorrow, for it is yet unborn." My sunrise pictures are so different from one another; you can hardly believe they are taken from the same tripod at the same time every morning over a period of a few months. They prove beyond reasonable doubt that every day is different than the one before and the one after. But they keep coming. The fact that I can take the next picture is so darn sweet. To welcome the new day, to celebrate its dawn, to diligently import the new pictures into my iPhoto library—what a kick!

In my humble opinion, for anybody, who has suffered from depression and insomnia, just looking at my pictures should suffice. Every person who went through even one single episode of depression for as little as a couple of weeks or a month, knows that the DIFFERENCE between SUNSET and SUNRISE is similar to the difference between life and death. Seriously, when I was severely depressed, I couldn't wait for the sun to set down, I wanted darkness, quiet, no life, no sounds, no birds, nothing. I wanted NOTHING please. I longed for nothingness. I would look at the clock and if it was 2 am or 3 am I would be: "Yeiii, thank God there are more hours of darkness ahead!" I dreaded the sunrise, the setting in of the new day. I was longing for the dark hours of the night. This book and these pictures are about waking up from this state and rising to discovery, to welcoming the light and the new daybreak, to anticipating the sunrise and to celebrating it. So, my beautiful pictures alone should be enough for you to lighten up a bit, no? Besides, they say that everyone should welcome the sunrise wherever he is and that morning meditations are best done at sunrise. If you can't catch it, they say, then meditate in front of a wallpaper with a beautiful sunrise, or choose a screen that has a gorgeous picture of a sunrise. Yeah, yeah, yeah, I know—repetitive, but true!!

The name of my new condominium is "Papillon Place" and it is a chapter of its own: "Planet Papillon". So much to tell (and show in pictures) about this place—but don't worry—thanks to cyber space—there are only links to my photo albums and you can check them out only if you want.

Further there are some of my most precious email exchanges which I grouped in the chapter "Eternal Emails". Here I had to deal with the anonymity issue since some of them are with my new friends from AA. I decided to give my friends numbers such as AA01, AA7, AA101 etc. for two main reasons: 1. It protects their anonymity (including their gender, although I thought of making women carry even numbers and men odd, surprise!!) and 2. When it comes to recovery from addiction of all sorts, I believe today what Melody Beattie writes in her book "Beyond Codependency" regarding proper attribution of ideas and theories to the appropriate sources: "Sometimes it's difficult to do that in the recovery field because many people say many of the same things." One thing is sure: "numbering" my brave heroes from AA in order to protect their anonymity made them even more particular and highly individual to me. They are by all means not "just numbers", not just another brick in the wall, please!—they stay put and are unforgettable, unrepeatable, irreplaceable and eternal to me.

Further in this modest booklet the reader will find the richest, most thoughtful and most responsible reference section on your self-help shelf. Here my academic background had to kick in. I am famous for mastering the secondary literature on the topic I am writing about like no one else. References upon request: ask my supervisor at the German Department of the University of Toronto. The chapter on the secondary literature of my doctoral dissertation was ACTUALLY quoted and praised in "Women for German" back in 2005. I am a diligent academic and the fear of plagiarism is my biggest nightmare—so I make sure I quote and quote and quote. And really: higher education doesn't make you KNOW everything, it rather teaches you where to LOOK for knowledge and information on a given topic. It lets you appreciate referring to other sources and so gives substance to your sharing of information and knowledge.

The biggest feature of this booklet remains its urgency. The need to put down in ONE BREATH my experience in the last six months is the reason for not editing this piece of writing and it is of course its biggest beauty. There are pages not even revisited since they have been written back in the fall of 2011. I just copied and pasted them for my final submission to iUniverse. Scrambled always in the wee hours of a true insomniac between 3 and 7 AM, not edited, disorganized, enraptured. That's what this booklet is all about. "To take off with all possible haste, as to intercept enemy aircraft" is one of the definitions of "scramble" in the free online dictionary. Exactly my case: I had finally recognized my new (old!) enemy and I wanted to fight back. I readily surrendered mentally to my condition, I admitted wholeheartedly that "Yes, I am an alcoholic"—step one of the 12 step program and I almost instantly declared war of life and death to my depression and alcoholism. I needed this aggression to be focused in the right direction. For the past six months I have been showing BOTH my middle fingers to EVERY LCBO or Beer store I pass by while driving. And this action is accompanied by the loudest cursing in the most obscene, awful, arrogant, dirty language you can ever imagine. It is very corporal and involves terrible details about private body parts and pivotal images. I address personally every bottle of vodka, gin, scotch, red and white wine produced on earth and send them to hell in the most explicit and profound manner possible. My cursing is extremely colorful and unheard of. Some store locations I had to revisit ON PURPOSE just to give myself the chance to spill my verbal shit all over them. Brrrrrr, scary and yet it feels sooo good. Sorry about this detour, but I STRONGLY recommend to you showing BOTH your middle fingers to the LCBO and to the Beer store if you are a recovering alcoholic: it is darn liberating and it feels terrific, trust me! The same goes to addicts of other substances. At least picture it in your mind: it would certainly supply you with so much power over the freaking bottles and chemicals, waiting patiently to be picked up by YOU from the shelf or from someone's "helping palm" and to be paid dearly for at the cashier and later you know where by YOU AND YOU A-L-O-N-E. And then inevitably—by anyone else you love and cherish.

I wrote "Good Midnight, Insomniacs" while anxiously awaiting to take pictures of the sunrise. I spilled my heart and soul and I couldn't care less about "literary" value. And, pardon my French, but all those "correct" prepositions in English! When you spot a grammar mistake here (and you will—like in Conan O'Brian's Monday night show, haaa) please do remember that I know (and teach) the absolute correct grammar of German and Russian—two much more tragically complicated languages, so give me a break in English, a language I acquired last in my life. That is just another disclaimer, okay? And if you need to know the truth, I like shopping in IKEA because all the instructions even for a can opener come sometimes in 30 languages (fact, I have proof!) and I keep these sheets in my bathroom with the magazines for myself and visitors to enrich their language knowledge while . . . There is also a notebook and a pen there for them to write down what is on their mind, but it has to be honest. So far, not too may entries. But the notebook IS there waiting and that is what counts. Just in case you are ready to share.

I wanted my booklet to be modest, sincere and crazy helpful! No big literary ambitions here. I kept thinking about the inscription on the triangle of my first AA desire chip: >RECOVERY< >UNITY< >SERVICE<. Service, service, service. I know it is the final step 12 of the program, I know I was just a few months into the program, but I needed to give back. It was time to pay back. It was time simply to be there. Be available. Speak. Help.

One morning I read again the letter I received from the Dean of the School for Graduate Studies at the University of Toronto after my Convocation as a PhD on June 1, 2005. I quote:

"Dear Dr. Alma Christova,

Please accept my warmest congratulations on the successful completion of all the requirements for the doctorate at the University of Toronto. You have identified a significant goal, and you have achieved it. The proud ritual of awarding doctoral degrees has been underway for over a century at the University of Toronto. I share with all those who have contributed to this institution's excellent programs, the hope that the opportunity for advanced study will benefit both our graduates and our world.

I sincerely hope that your doctoral degree marks both the achievement of a personal goal and a commitment to social responsibility and leadership, wherever life may take you.

Sincerely yours,
/sgd., ill./
Susan Pfeiffer,
Dean."

I attached a photo of this letter in the Appendix. Who knew that ACDC, AA and all my other self-help groups would be my field and vocation where life actually took me? No one. I—the least.

So here comes my actual warning to you, my dear Reader. I have to seriously warn you that (luckily!!) my booklet ended up containing some extraordinary valuable insights here and there and also some surprisingly moving chapters, so I strongly suggest that you skip skipping pages and your best bet remains to read the whole thing in order not to miss anything that speaks to you, could significantly improve your own recovery and tends to be important in general. The table of content is very approximate: as an academic I know that "it is all in the name" and a good definition means everything, but the titles of my chapters are really randomly chosen and you might find something in the conclusion that actually belongs in the introduction and vice versa. Unedited, remember? Just bear with me and keep reading. Once we have established that I am crazy and that's a given, it's a big relief for both sides: reader and writer. It's nothing ground-breaking really, but it's fresh and sincere and it comes from the first-hand experience of yet another recovering (but now "DIScovering!!) addict.

This modest booklet is also about turning frustration into power and strength. Turning your wildest shortcomings into your most powerful weapons. You need to be HEAVILY armed in your war with depression and addiction, there is no doubt about that in my mind today.

When Whitney Houston died on February 11, 2012 at the age of 48 in the bath tab of a hotel in Los Angeles and coincidentally the same day my publishing co-ordinator Mars at iUniverse said "NO MORE drafts, Alma, send your final version now!" I grasped for the millionth time in a row: no matter who you are, how talented, rich or poor, black or white, addiction wants your life.

Addiction wants you dead. Period. Get armed then, declare your war with your addiction please. It's simply a war of life and death. YOU NEED TO STAY ALIVE.

Here is the link to my sunrise pictures:
http://pix.kg/p/1936562041105%3A315883704/scl

ACKNOWLEDGEMENTS

This is another wrong "chaptering". As you have seen in the 'Author's Warning', it is anything but that. One can think that I have no idea what genre is. Not so. Let's agree that my chapters are some sort of essays? Here for instance you will find me talking about the people who are on my mind. Who I kept in mind while scrambling these notes and whom this booklet is written for after all. As Marquez said about the critics of "One Hundred Year of Solitude", I paraphrase: "I have no idea what these people are finding in my book and how they come up with their analyses. All I did was a joke between me and the people who are close to me."

    I want to thank my son Chris for taking our traditional two-month summer trip to Bulgaria without me last summer. In 21 years this was his first time alone in Sofia and we have spent 207 days apart. When my husband Andy and I took him to the airport on June 22, 2011 and waved goodbye at him, I was full of fear that I won't make it to see him again. My depression was at its absolute worst on that Wednesday afternoon, driving back home in my husband's truck (and company). Deadly silence, stupid traffic, big knot in my throat, never ending longest day of the year. To close this most painful cycle quickly let me report that meeting Chris upon his arrival back in Toronto on Monday January 16, 2012 is one of the five biggest triumph moments in my life so far. He was paramountly embarrassed of course, because the screaming, the jumping, the laughing, the crying, the absolute crazy reaction on my part was well registered and witnessed by everybody in the arrival hall of Pearson's Terminal 1. Hahaaa. Victory, victory, ultimate victory: the biggest prey of my life was back in my arms. And I was alive to live it. These ten enraptured minutes are an all-important milestone in my recovery—the heaviest chip I received so far for staying sober and keeping in the game. The contrast between June 22, 2011 and January 16, 2012 is best described in pictures. As always. (Please see the Appendix). Chris knew that I have become a warrier after he left—I called him overseas at least once a day 207 times—now he registered my victories and realized that I had won quite a few major battles in my on-going war against addiction. He saw me marching (LOUD) on a new path.

I am grateful to my current husband Andy for letting me go on July 25, 2011. It made all the difference between life and death. We both know that for a fact today. And we both know today that our inferiorities can never be satisfied by any one but ourselves. Andy has been great to all my cars and to all technology problems I ever encountered and which needed a solution fast. He likes (and knows) boats and other gadgets and his garage is his paradise. When I was kicked out to smoke there in the winter months, it seemed like a 'Folterraum' for me—full of inquisition tools and danger.

Special thanks to my friends from the Bulgarian artists gang in Toronto for their love and for their art. Vacnche's "Well under the Red", "Father Freud and Almichka", "Tulips", "Sleeping Beauty", all the graphics and caricatures have been living with me in Planet Papillon as a strong connection with my past and a voiced reminder of AA's slogan 'Remember when'. Rosita's "Country Road, "Lighthouse in the Sun" and especially "The Wave" are symbols of my very first steps on a road never traveled before. George's "Jazzman and a Rooster" just celebrates the fun in life. I am still waiting for a painting from George No. 2. Hahaaaa.

My talented graphic designer Djema is an Apple pro and the best massage-master in the world. She kept an eye on me during the darkest days of my depression, often knocking on our front door yelling that she is sick and tired of me not picking up the phone and let's have a cigarette immediately! Thank you, Jeto, for so many things—giving me books, sharing your own (huge) experience, and not least for coming to

Family Day in my Day Treatment Program at ACDC and so saving my participation and keeping me in! In the Appendix there are pictures of you, I hope you don't mind the publicity. Thank you, Sofi, for restoring our friendship after three long years when it was fractured and needed a patient rehabilitation. Owning an all-successful air-conditioning business, you surely know how to fuel back warmth in my once frosted veins like no one else I've met in Canada. And your new cat kills me: she is so fat that petting her feels like touching wood.

The Markov's family in Thessaloniki, Greece: Milena has been my ultimate inspiration ever since she was born in 1965. She is my first cousin and we are daughters of two sisters. Each of us has one brother and we are more like sisters than first cousins. Our mutual friends swear to God that we are so alike in the way we speak, they can hardly tell the difference on the phone. We grew up in our maternal grandmother's house and share a fabulous relationship. Milena is the most witty person I know. Our email exchange over the years since I left Bulgaria is a bestseller in the making. She saved my life on numerous occasions during periods of dark depression and despair. Milena ALWAYS stood by me and she always will. She knows too well that I am not able to ever thank her properly, so Musi, just keep being! Her husband Jordan (whom I introduced to Milena in 1985—you are welcome, Danka!) is a Sorbonne graduate in Sociology and a talented artist. Attached in the Appendix is a link to a photo album of his paintings. He only started painting later in life while Milena was persistently feeding the entire family thanks to her many talents and language proficiency. Nowadays they both celebrate life in a perfect harmony when it comes to marriage. They have millions of friends and usually have visitors all the time in Thessaloniki. When it's time for a vacation in the summer, at Easter or at Christmas, their unique cottage in Ribaritsa—in the heart of the beautiful Balkan Mountains—becomes the center of the universe. Everybody wants to be there. Their two children—my niece Dima and my nephew Jordan Jr.—are my solid connection with the 21st century and its technology. We live online together and they make most of my days by sharing links on Facebook or emailing me. Well, there is also Dima's dissertation finished in January this year and submitted as a requirement for her Diploma in Fashion Journalism from the University in Epsom, England which she dedicated to . . . . ME!! This rocked my Cosmos big time. It is entitled "Language is more powerful than we think, but can we think without a language? Throughout time numerous celebrated philosophers and linguists have explored the relation of language to the thought of its speakers, and the debate still continues today. To what extent does language influence thought?" How about that? And it's brilliantly written, too. I still have to figure out why Dima dedicated it to me, but let me assure you that opening her manuscript has left me speechless. I still stick to my old recipe: in order to serve a well done foreign language you need to cook your mother tongue to perfection. To a future full of funny words, Dima, in all the languages we speak! Thank you again, Sweetheart, you really made my year! Knowing that I have a DIRECT impact on you two being born in the first place, (yes, Danka Sr., we know you owe me big time for your wife and for your kids), I arrogantly consider you and Dani Jr. my own co-creation and blatantly share the pride and joy of your existence with your parents and the world.

On the European shore there are many other people to acknowledge and to thank, but let me BOLDLY point out a person who LITERALLY kept me above water in the period of highest risk of my depression and addiction: the entire 2010 and the first half of 2011: Lusi Mindova and her family. There are pictures of Lusi in the Appendix and once you have a look at her, you already know what I am talking about. There is such a harmony between the inside and the outside. I owe Lusi surviving July and August 2010 in Bulgaria: she fed me, she found a psychiatrist to help me, her husband drove me to appointments and their cottage in Izvor was a safety island. Thank you both so much, Lusi and Rumi! And my other special Rumi Popova: you are the only relative of mine who has sent us greeting cards for Christmas, Easter, all our birthdays, anniversaries and the precious "martenichki" EVERY single year since I immigrated—no exception for now over twenty years.

INTRODUCTION

"We are all insane, but some are overdoing it."
Dr. Hristo Hristov

My name is Alma. (About time, no?) I am an insomniac (like you), probably bipolar (so far I managed to get into serious professional and personal conflict at least four psychiatrists in Toronto and Sofia), and a menopausal (ouch) discovering alcoholic (as of today I am considered "a shining beacon of recovery" in my Alcoholics Anonymous home group in Mississauga). On Sunday, March 25, 2012 I will receive my First Year Sobriety Medallion. The inscription will read DUM SPIRO SPERO (from Latin: "As long as I breathe, I hope"). I will report to you in another letter how did it go. I am totally hyper, although I have a few accomplishments which came with gold medals. But this compares to nothing.

I am born and bred in beautiful Bulgaria and Dr. Hristo Hristov is my one and only brother: a talented psychiatrist and a devoted alcoholic. I am his most difficult case ever since he graduated from medical school while for me he is the best psychotherapist in the world: a born genius in disguise. He is five years older than me and one of my earliest memories of him involves him reading with a flashlight under his bed cover. In my humble estimate, Izi has read more books than anyone I know. And no matter how hard he tries to drown his intellect and personality in booze, he still surfaces as the funniest guy for me.

In my precious country of origin Alcoholics Anonymous is not an active organization yet. Do Bulgarians need AA? Do Bulgarian men and women of all ages have problems with alcohol, drugs, concurrent mental disorders and addictions in general? You bet! You guys know who you are, you are my most precious lunatics and you (and I) hold on vice better than anyone I've met in my 30 cosmopolitan years of traveling and immigration. Proud to be Bulgarian? No doubt. The only Bulgarian proverb quoted on page 78 in my edition of The Little ZEN Companion goes like this: "If you wish to drown, don't torture yourself with shallow waters". How cool is that? I mean 'cool' as 'scary and dear'.

But since July last year I rapidly and steadily started to thank God every single day for probably the only good thing I did while drinking heavily back in the 90ies: immigrating to Canada. Here AA is prominent and stable. As my friend AA007 says, now I have no choice but to translate the "Big Book" into Bulgarian, retire from University of Toronto and the Ministry of the Attorney General of Ontario, pack some brochures and fly overseas to organize the first AA group in Sofia.

And, why not?

To qualify as an alcoholic? Okay, to put it clearly, I wrote this booklet as a continuation to one particular letter of gratitude.

On August 12, 2011 I graduated from the three-week intensive Day Treatment Program for outpatients at the Addictions and Concurrent Disorders Centre in Credit Valley Hospital in Mississauga, Ontario. On my way home that Friday afternoon I felt the compelling urge to express in writing the profound effect this educational course had on me. More importantly, I hastened to address the CEO of the hospital from a patient's point of view in regards with preserving such initiatives* since we were told over the course of the program that the Centre's existence was threatened by budget considerations and hospital merges. Later in the evening I wrote the four pages long recommendation letter to Dr. John Smith in one breath and mailed it first thing next Saturday morning.

The problem was that I could not ACTUALLY stop writing this letter. I would be thinking about it all the time, taking it with me to places I go, talking about it with everybody—my son Chris and my husband Andy, my relatives, my colleagues, my friends here and overseas, my neighbors, bankers, dentists, opticians, sales persons, at AA meetings, any strangers I would spend more than 5 minutes no matter where I've met them. I started taking notes while driving, the former 'drinking and driving' became 'driving and writing', then later in November it escalated to 'driving and taking pictures'. I kept a notebook and a pencil in the bathroom, talking to myself and what not. Yes, you guessed it: I got obsessed with it. I would find no peace unless I wrote it down. I didn't think of any therapeutical value, of any release, of any catharsis. I just kept writing, with no editing, no breaks. As a recovering (and menopausal—ouch) alcoholic and a patient diagnosed with a clean-cut case of "severe clinical depression" as recently as July 14 2011, I welcomed this new cross-addiction: it kicked me out of bed at 4 AM the latest every morning. My bed was the place I would spend 16-18 hours a day in the last three years. "Sleeping" wouldn't describe this state properly. By June this year it felt more like a grave or a coffin at best. Today I call it my "narcotic" bed and at times of total physical and mental exhaustion I kindly ask my husband Andy for permission to take a nap there in order to recuperate. I sleep there like nowhere else on earth. Thankfully, Andy is generous and lets me do it.

So here in front of you is the expansion of my letter of gratitude to Dr. Smith. Can you imagine him receiving that piece of writing in his mail? I am sure he is obliged to read reference letters from patients. I am sure that he enjoys reading letters of gratitude. What would he think of me? Hmmm, I don't want to know. But in case I am wrong about Dr. Smith, I will send him a copy of this booklet.

In any case, it became a matter of life and death for me to share my experience since July last year with as many insomniacs and all sorts of mental disorders victims as possible. My family and friends have their ears full by now. I am unstoppable in talking and emailing, skyping, facebooking and all else. Unless I published my story, I couldn't find peace. I have met over 350 NEW people in the past six months. Here I count people whose name(s) I know, who know my name and we are in touch in one way or another. I owe my SINCERE gratitude to almost all of them for simply existing at this particular time and for the sheer fact that our roads crossed. They have to remain anonymous of course, and they will stay anonymous, although in the process of writing I developed second thoughts regarding anonymity both in AA and when it comes to mental health issues in general. More about that in my conclusion, here it should suffice to say, that today I feel like SCREAMING LOUD and CLEAR when it comes to the traditionally idiotic stigma that surrounds depression and mental health issues. North America (and of course Eastern Europe) of the 21st century are witnessing a PANDEMIC in mental health problems. What are both "continents" doing about it? They keep quite. Silence and ignorance, impatience, fear, superstition and often disgust are the typical inherited gut reaction to such problems. I have a lot to say not only about the public (kept in the dark), but especially about general practitioners, family doctors, nurses etc. I get upset already!! So, you will find more on that topic later. For now let's park the idea: Enough bullshit!

My Life Story for AA

DUM SPIRO SPERO
(From Latin: As long as I breathe, I hope)

I was born on Sunday May 15, 1960 in Sofia, Bulgaria. My Mom was a pediatrician and my Dad was an engineer. I have one older brother Hristo who is a psychiatrist. Both my Mom and my brother are alcoholics. My maternal grandfather was an alcoholic as well. My Dad never developed a drinking problem but drank "responsibly" on all occasions our family hosted or attended.

Alcohol is a big part of our culture—when we grew up there was a party almost every weeknight and definitely a couple of gatherings on the weekend with a lot of booze around. The choice was mainly hard liquor such as rakia, (schnapps or brandy), vodka, ouzo as starters or aperitifs, followed by tones of beer, red or white wine. Let's not forget how affordable alcohol was in the sixties and seventies in the Eastern Communist Block. In Bulgaria 1 liter of Russian vodka for example would cost 1-2 Levs, i.e. 0,5-1 CAD.

I remember being offered on a regular basis a glass of red wine mixed with sprite at home as early as at the age of 14-15. My family used to say: "It is better to have ONE glass at home at Sunday lunch or dinner than MANY outside with strangers . . ."

My teen years were marked by my Mom's increasing drinking problem. My brother started drinking heavily in the army (i.e. 18-20 when I was respectively 13-15) and it became awful when he returned home—with my Dad we had to cope both with my Mom's and my brother's drinking. There was a special bond between my Dad and me at that time, which I later in life registered between my son and my second husband. From today's point of view I know now that we must have become co-dependent. My brother continued to drink heavily through his medical school, his two marriages and basically until this day. He is 56 now. Both my parents passed away—my Dad in 1997 and my Mom in 2008. She never sobered up. I received the call on Saturday November 1, 2008 while getting ready for my Saturday German School. It was All Saints' Day in Bulgaria. The morning after Halloween. She died in her sleep like only saints do.

It is important to mention that I was aware of the effects of alcohol and was clear about alcoholism being a disease at a very early age since my family has at least two medical doctors in each generation. I knew at least part of it involves genetic predisposition and was warned to be affected by it both from an intellectual point of view and by first hand experience witnessing my Mom's and my brother's progression.

I first got drunk in high school. It was a German immersion school, which I attended between 14 and 19 years of age. It was in my senior years where my drinking became visible to my classmates and myself. It was self explanatory that we would drink at home: birthday parties, outside in the park, during vacation camps and especially during "brigades"—the one summer month you spend in the country as a high school student working for the government picking whatever—apples, tomatoes, cucumbers, corn, etc. We didn't get paid for this work. It was obligatory to attend. We were fed and had a place to sleep. Looked a bit like being in the army. I started smoking cigarettes relatively "late"—in my fourth year, but became a chain-smoker almost immediately. Price of a pack—30 cents. I nevertheless managed to graduate being awarded a Gold Medal for Academic Achievement.

During my entire 5 years of high school I was involved in competitive swimming and played a lot of table tennis. The last three years in a row

I even became the girl's high school champion and our team of three girls was three times champion among all Foreign language immersion schools in the city of Sofia!!

In 1979—immediately after high school—I continued my education in German Studies first at the University of Sofia and then at Humboldt University in Berlin, which at this point of time was the capital of the German Democratic Republic.

I never quit smoking and my alcohol intake increased severely during these 5 years, especially in Germany. I thought I couldn't handle the stress of being away from home. From today's point of view, I probably was very depressed for the first time in my life, but couldn't recognize the signs. I thought it was nostalgia. I was home sick and drank like a fish to handle it. Upon my return to Bulgaria I got married to an alcoholic in 1986. We drank and drank and drank together . . . We were functioning alcoholics and continued to work.

In 1988 my husband was sent to Helsinki Finland to work as a Station Manager for Balkan Airlines. We stayed in Scandinavia for 5 years. Five long, dark, cold winters. Looking back at this time I realize—TODAY—that this was the first time in my life where I experienced a severe depression, again unrecognized and not treated. We drank non-stop.

My son Chris was born on March 13, 1990. I quit smoking and drinking for three years. I thought I was cured and had the time of my life being a mother. I stayed at home these three years and only gave private German lessons to some pretty rhapsodic Finns.

In 1993 my husband got promoted to a General Manager position with Balkan Airlines and was transferred to Toronto to open a charter operation. We moved in the summer. Chris started kindergarten because my husband wanted me to work with him in the office as a reservation supervisor and admin assistant, basically as his secretary and slave. He said he wouldn't trust anybody else. I took the job. On the first day after work I relapsed. Started to drink more than before. But somehow didn't start smoking again. Kept my job.

Three years later we got divorced and my ex-husband returned to Europe. I quit drinking immediately and this time—the summer of 1996—a monstrous depression hit me. I struggled between going back to Bulgaria and staying in Canada. I decided to immigrate with my son—6 years old at the time and started my PhD program at UofT. I was a single mother for 5 years. I was in school, Chris started elementary school. I was sober during the entire period but never got rid of my depression which now presented itself as SAD (Seasons Affected Disorder)—I would go to Bulgaria in the summer and be happy and then returning in September it would be hell until Christmas. Then March comes—I'll be okay again until September. My brother started to voice his concerns about these obvious cycles, but I handled them somehow. Again, I was not treated for any mental disorders at this time. My social life was exceptionally beautiful during these years. I was involved in my studies, I was teaching three nights a week, I had a lot of friends, I was very active in my son's school, and we traveled extensively. I managed to keep busy, did a lot of exercise and made a significant progress in my graduate program accomplishing all the requirements in a very short period of time. I had my entire course work done, passed my comprehensive exams and all that was left was to write and defend my dissertation.

But the new Millennium brought me a new husband. My son Chris was ten years old. I remarried on Canada Day July 1, 2000, had our honeymoon in Bulgaria in August and on the way back I had a miscarriage. I was hospitalized for a couple of days and on the way home from St. Michael's hospital I asked my husband to stop at the LCBO and to buy me one liter of vodka "Finlandia", which I trusted religiously and of which my liver has probably processed a full tank in Helsinki. I had my first drink in the car after 5 years of abstinence. The distance between the store and our condominium in Harbour Square is about 300 m. Needless to say, this nanosecond became problematic as it happened. My new husband never saw me drinking in the brief period of our dating and up to this moment. Chris was 5 when I quit the previous time, so wouldn't have had some vivid memories of a drunk mother as I did of mine, but it was all gone within the blink of an eye.

Did it become problematic right away? You bet. I know today that relapse brings you back to the very first sober day of your sober period no matter how long it was—a month, a year, a decade or 25 years. It is, as you have never stopped. Someone said in an AA meeting lately that if you don't work on your "actual" recovery during abstinent periods, your addiction is quietly doing push-ups while you don't drink and waits patiently for your relapse. How sad is that? How about THAT, really . . .

The fall of 2000 became immediate hell. Chris was in school, my husband Andy was working all day, I was supposed to write my thesis at home or in the library and I was stripped from all work obligations outside the apartment. Without having to even leave the building, I could still shuttle between the pool and the sauna, the squash room, the table tennis room, the billiard room, the gym, the party room, the book club, the many free classes in Yoga, Pilates, dancing, playing bridge two times a week, seeing my friends on the weekends, cooking beautiful meals for my family etc. But what did I do? You know what I did. I immobilized and imprisoned myself. I didn't go to the library, I stopped shopping and cooking, I stopped picking up the mail from downstairs and I drank. All day long. By the time my boys were home, I would be asleep. I didn't write a word. Stopped picking up the phone. I started to vanish.

The confusion in Chris and Andy was enormous. This is the time of their biggest bonding actually—they got scared together and this fear connected them in a way, which nothing can alter even today.

AGAIN—I didn't seek help. Talked regularly to my family overseas, including my Mom and my brother who had their own difficulties fighting alcoholism. I started to lye in ways, which produced nightmares of unseen brutality. Weeks were passing, Then months. It got worse in a startling progression.

The wake up call came in June 2001—I received a phone call that my Mom is diagnosed with breast cancer and I needed to go home immediately. They called one day before her operation. All three of us packed and left: within 24 hours we were in Bulgaria. I was a mess.

I have wasted the past 10 months in drinking, jeopardized my studies, my marriage, my parenting, my friends, my social network, have been risking my life on a daily basis. I'll never forget my Mom's expression when she saw me entering her room in the hospital. Above everything in her face there was guilt. There was no way to convince her that this was not her fault. I learned later how excruciating this feeling was. But I didn't want her to feel that way, so I stopped drinking again. Cold turkey as usual. AGAIN I shocked my body and my brain by throwing myself into withdrawal of unfelt severity. At this point I realized how big my problem was.

The summer was over, my Mom recovered and we headed back to Toronto, to the fall and to reality.

With the help of my husband and the love of my son I stayed sober for the next 4 years. I finished my dissertation, defended on December 14, 2004 with honors. Took me twice the time because I returned to teaching. I divided my time between full time teaching classes at UofT and writing my dissertation, so it took double the time. From today's point of view I am grateful, because it meant two extra years of sobriety.

By now you should be able to trace the pattern? What happened after my defense? Yes, that's right: on Christmas Day 2004 when celebrating my Doctorate and my son's name day with the entire world, I relapsed after 4 years of total abstinence and sobriety.

This time in this brief fast-paced week between Christmas and New Year I literally lost my mind. Physically, emotionally, mentally and intellectually I hit rock bottom within hours. The impact was out of this world. Within 7 days of constant binging I terminated everything positive and welcomed a hell of negativity. I lost control so rapidly that I quit my teaching job for the winter term between January and April 2005 only hours after being given an additional course, which was meant to give me more recognition and more money. I packed and left on my own to Bulgaria for a month leaving behind Chris in grade 9 in a horrible high school and Andy to take care of him and to work in the middle of the winter. As far as irrational thinking, irrational behaviour and irrational decision-making goes, I produced a catastrophe. In terms of a relapse, it tasted more as a suicide.

I thought I am getting psychotic or bipolar at best. My brother confirmed the diagnosis. They were worried sick. I have spent most of January in Bulgaria in bed, unable to function, totally depressed, flat as an automobile tire. I realized what I have done: I have lost my job at UofT, lost my income for the rest of the year, and abandoned my son and my husband for no particular reason. There was no logic in my actions, no rational explanation of this behaviour. And needless to say, upon my return in February, I didn't feel welcomed by my husband. Or wanted, or loved. Something has happened that I couldn't repair anymore.

Although I was able to get my job back in 2006 and even got a second job as a court interpreter for the Ministry of the Attorney General of Ontario in the spring of the same year, ever since my Defense party on Christmas Day 2004 nothing could change for the better. I tried the so called geographical move. We moved to Mississauga in the fall of 2006. This time my depression brought me to a doctor. The isolation of the new place was undescribable. We lived in a huge empty house, my friends from downtown claimed that they don't have visa for Mississauga and cannot cross the Humber River, I needed to drive hundreds of kilometers a day to get to work in courthouses all over the province—Ottawa, and Windsor to mention a couple—I didn't know anybody in Lorne Park and I wanted to die. I HAD to seek professional medical care. My choice of psychiatrist was a very poor one. Actually, I had NO choice and this is going to be discussed AT length later in my book, because only now I realize how problematic the situation with mental health treatment for Canadians, or at least for Ontarians and Torontonians IS!!! (Today I consider it A CRIME!!!—more later in my chapter on Medical Help!!) To make a long story short: on November 7, 2006 I was prescribed antidepressants for the first time in my life.

I started taking Cipralex (SSRI). Things were getting worse, because I couldn't stop drinking. This continued for the next 4 years.

I hit rock bottom on Christmas 2010. My favorite niece Boryana came for a visit. It took her 40 hours to arrive in Toronto due to snow storms in Sofia and Frankfurt am Main. It was my dream to have her here ever since I immigrated in Canada. She got the visa and her brother Ivan (Abo) bought the high season expensive airline ticket. She was supposed to stay for three weeks between December 20, 2010 and January 5, 2011. What did I do? I was drinking from 6 AM and stayed in bed most of the time, constantly intoxicated. She packed and left a week after she arrived and 10 days before planned. I couldn't drive her to the airport because I was very drunk at 12 noon on December 27, 2010. She was extremely upset with me and couldn't wait to call a cab, headed to the bus stop on our street in Cedarglen Gate, I followed her in my pajamas and begged her to stay. She got on the bus and when I lost sight of it, I returned home to my grave-bed and checked online the lethal dose of all medications I had at home and can say that for the first time in my life I got serious suicidal thoughts. The picture on my front cover is taken at 12.22 pm on December 27, 2010 from my bedroom window and shows the bus stop where I lost Buba a few minutes prior to taking it. It was taken with the same camera I am taking my sunrise pictures today. It shows PRECISELY what I was feeling: frosted. I felt for the first time what it means when it's said "the blood froze in my veins." Buba left behind all the gifts she received, first and foremost her "Arrival-to-Canada-Flower", which then became "The Flower Left Behind" in my photo-album "Remember when". The days and weeks since that day were spent as a zombie in a deep thick fog. I was sleepwalking during the day and having nightmares during the night. My son said to me: "I see you vanishing, I WANT to help you and I can't and that is killing me." This coming from him, who also took the family tradition road and is studying Athletic Therapy in Sheridan College, having lost or disappointed my ENTIRE family here and back home in Bulgaria, this time I felt I had to choose between life and death. For real.

I didn't want to kill my son. That was the last thing I wanted to do on earth. I felt my Mom's guilt. It became unbearable.

So my last drink was on March 18, 2011—Friday—at 7.30 PM (approximately) from a bottle of Johnny Walker which I opened in the morning and kept all day in the wardrobe of my bedroom. It was almost finished, but I remember "symbolically" pouring the last 50-100 ml in the bathroom sink.

The withdrawal was worse than ever. I started taking antidepressants again right away. This time the side effects were brutal.

I had to seek help because I felt that this is pretty much my last chance. I was extremely lucky to join the Day Treatment Program of the Centre for Addictions and Concurrent Disorders at Credit Valley Hospital in Mississauga. I owe the contact to my friend AA01, who accidentally mentioned the Centre during an AA meeting I attended in February 2011 in Port Credit while still drinking. This is miracle Number One in my recovery. When I called her to let her know that I graduated from Stage 1 on November 23, 2011 and thanked her for showing me my "North Star", she cried on the phone. She is a young, robust, black girl with a pearl smile and she is my ultimate Mother Mary.

Later the therapists in ACDC referred me to more self-help groups such as Stepping Stones, Women for Sobriety, Dual Recovery Anonymous, Equilibrium etc. Even if I learned something from my previous sobriety periods, I have to say that with age everything gets much more difficult. If I want to carry a message it would be to young people and to prevention: I decided to be honest especially with my students at UofT and I admitted that I am a chronic alcoholic who FINALLY decided to conquer my addiction by staying sober for the rest of my life and to put all my efforts in a lasting (and not least exemplary) recovery. I realized that making some major mistakes is the rightest thing we can achieve in life, but REPEATING them senseless can and will be fatal. Whitney Houston's case is one of a full blown chronic pathological addiction, treated THREE times in rehabilitation centres where nothing was objectively achieved, and she was STILL testing her physical strength during her last week prior to the Grammy Awards. As always, death makes our awareness of life so acute. I am sure that over the same weekend there were thousands of people all over the world who lost their lives to addiction, prescription drugs, painkillers abuse, drugs and alcohol. We need to remember that our bodies can take only that much abuse.

I cannot stop repeating what I learned in ACDC: The most important objective in recovery is to look for underlying mental conditions. The root, the primary cause is often a mental disorder and alcoholism is a secondary self-medicating attempt. And the absolute must: I will break my anonymity in order to give an example of courage and success in recovery. Recovery> Service> Unity—the triangle of AA is on my silver ring which replaced my wedding ring on October 1, 2011 at the Annual AA Round Up at the Ukrainian Church in Cawthra Road in Mississauga.

And finally, the new knowledge of my situation brings me back to a thought I've read in a book called "Writing outside the Nation" by Turkish-American writer Azade Seyhan: "It is a truism born of the idea of paradigm shift that when the present changes, so does the past. When a new structure of knowledge emerges, our understanding of the past often undergoes a radical revision."

That is to say that my life story today is much different from my life story if I had to write it back in 1990 or in 2000. That is all good news. It reminds me of reading "Gone with the Wind" at the age of twenty, then thirty, then forty and now fifty: I have read four different books. I hope that this time my own story will turn out with a happy end.

In AA's "Big Book" there is a case of a gentleman in his 60-ies who explained his joining AA at this relatively later stage of his life as follows: "I've come to realize that I can not hope for a brand new beginning of my life at 60. But I knew that I can hope for a much better ending." (goosebumps . . . .) PRECISELY! EXACTLY! DARN RIGHT! Just nailed it! Dead on! I still shiver remembering the profound effect this line had on me. That was 1000% what I was intuitively seeking as well. I didn't want to die drunk or depressed at 51 and leave my son with such a horrible legacy. I wanted to be his great, wonderful mother, a woman he can be proud of, the strongest example of recovery, an inspiring parent, a devoted friend and his favorite comedian. I wanted to achieve and be all that to Chris for even the shortest time and then die in peace. I needed badly to better the ending of my life and to improve dramatically my legacy. And of course—now that I am working on bettering the ending of my life, it took me by NO SURPRISE to witness how many new beginnings this involves. On a daily basis. Today every invitation turns into a new experience and most of the time into a precious memory. Mindfulness. Compassion. Love. (Take a picture!!) To be honest, today I feel that I am actually capable of reaching not only a better ending of my life, but even the BEST possible. Why not? What a thrill that is!!

DUM SPIRO SPERO

My ACDC Experience

Finally diagnosed as bipolar—the happiest day in my life!!

In this chapter I will share with you my personal experience at ACDC. I will let you know what I learned there and what they have taught us in case you cannot become an outpatient in their program. I will give you examples of my biggest mistakes until I got there.

You know, there is a Bulgarian proverb which goes around the idea that smart people learn from their own mistakes, but smarter people learn from other people's mistakes. Yes, that is prevention indeed. I want to share my mistakes with you so that you don't have to repeat them marching on your path.

As a very dear friend of mine has put in one of her many precious emails to me: "Sometimes we dread life, sometimes we overestimate it."

In my group at ACDC we started the program as eleven clients and stayed eleven—what an achievement!!

The staff called us 'clients', I thought I am a 'patient'.

Here is the letter I wrote to the CEO of Credit Valley Hospital on August 12, 2011—my Graduation Day from Stage 1 of the Day Treatment Program of ACDC:

12 August 2011
Mississauga

Dear Dr. Smith,

    I am one of eleven proud men and women, who graduated today from Stage 1 of the Day Treatment Program at the Addictions and Concurrent Disorders Centre in your hospital. Presently we are all entitled and enrolled in the Aftercare program of sixteen weeks. We are scheduled to accomplish this part of the program by November 30, 2012.

    I hasten to share with you the outcome of my program and the profound effect it had on ALL of us.

    Mental illnesses, addictions and drug abuse became pandemic in today's world and age. North America's first decade of the 21 century proved to be most challenging in this regard.

    Upon entering the program on Monday July 25, 2011 as participants with various addictions and concurrent disorders, we almost immediately came to realize that the medical treatment we have been receiving so far was borderline criminal at best. Most of us were familiar with AA, N/A, Al-Anon and other forms of self-help therapy and group support and as a matter of fact the majority of us are members of one group or another, but in all cases—regardless of our background and history of addiction—the professional MEDICAL treatment of our conditions was lacking or extremely poor. Today we know that underlying the alcohol (or narcotics) or any substance abuse there is an existent mental or emotional disorder, invisible to us, not known, a condition that only a specialist can diagnose. This medical care was MISSING in ALL of our cases. Most of us have suffered from their particular CHRONIC conditions over years, sometimes decades. Some had shorter experience as far as time is concerned, but at the time of the program's commencing we were ALL in a DEEP (LIFE-THREATENING) CRISIS spread over several months prior to July 2011.

This is when we came across the Day Treatment Program at ACDC in your hospital. Some voluntarily, some not so much voluntarily. Being covered by the OHIP was a crucial point of departure because most of us cannot afford financially other options. We took the necessary steps to be assessed and admitted as soon as possible. What we didn't know then—let's say in February this year, is that we encountered a chance of a life-time. We now feel extremely privileged and lucky to be the "chosen ones". This is a cliché and it tells the truth exactly as it is: This Program saved our lives. We are only now beginning to recover, but we are not dead—a very valid risk wasn't it for the Program.

In the process of the three weeks of intensive day care it became apparent, it became EYE-OPENING how huge the scope of mental health issues is. We realized that so many people who are suffering are unable to receive medical help. We realized that our GPs are either uneducated in the field of addiction and concurrent disorders, or simply corrupt to help us in this respect. They would prescribe antidepressant drugs with no mentioning of the dangers of drinking alcohol with it. Or in the "best" cases (like my own psychiatrist at the time) they would suggest "one drink only". Well, one drink is a very relative term to most people, but to alcoholics it is allowing a 'go ahead', a 'free ticket', a 'green light', because to alcoholics one drink can easily mean a whole bottle of hard liquor.

Realizing the critical mass of people affected by this neglect, we are determined to bring it to your attention, dear Dr. Smith. The quality of the program's organization, the competence and the integrity of the ENTIRE staff, the athmosphere turned out to be way beyond our highest expectations. On day one we were warmly welcomed "to a new home" and this promise did materialize. Every minute of the time of the therapists counted. Their every word did count. We were further urged to join and to continue to attend self-help group meetings and by "signing" our attendance sheets, this became a very important component of our recovery. Long time members of AA or NA finally "got the message" and started working the proverbial 12 steps programs for the first time in years. They realized that sometimes five or ten years of abstinence have past without one single hour of recovery. Newcomers found a new hope.

We promise on our part to do 100% of what is required to get better on our journey to wellbeing. But we need your expertise and good will as professionals to compass us, to teach us the tools and the coping mechanisms from a medical point of view in order to succeed. So we urge you to expand this program, forget cutting budgets due to hospital merges.

As we learned, we needed to return to the "circle of life" in order to cure ourselves. It was imperative to change. In North America of the 21st century most of us live in what Charlotte Kasl coined as "societal linear conciousness": We stand in a row, shoulder to shoulder, looking forward. We don't see the person next to us. We are unable to connect. Group therapy with its diacritical circle showed us that when we link our hands in a circle, we have a chance. Every link is as strong as the chain. And if someone falls, we see it, we feel it and we know it. And we can try to help him save himself. Isolation is deadly.

Please help more people join that circle. Let us quote: "The Vision of the Credit Valley Hospital is to be the finest hospital in Canada in the hearts and minds of the people we serve." Your Mission reads further: "The Credit Valley Hospital offers quality compassionate health care to the people of the growing communities of Peel and Halton."

Let us assure you once more that the staff at ACDC is taking both the Vision and the Mission of your Hospital beyond the highest expectations and dreams of both employers and patients.

With warm wishes,
Alma Christova

P.S. THANK YOU Dr. Jovey, Dr. Dayal, Jean, Angie, Declan, Michelle, Jacky, Alison and Virginia, what a blessing it is that you have chosen this profession!!

With you always,
Alma C.

(The name of the CEO is NOT Dr. Smith, of course.)

HIGHLIGHTS OF THE PROGRAM

1. The Three Headed Dragon

Nothing rocked me so deeply as the concept of the 'Three Headed Dragon' (and the DVD we were shown) as the VERY FIRST module of the program on Monday July 25, 2011. I have so many images of this (now favorite) 'beast' ever since and they are everywhere in my place as a reminder, including all the temporary kids' tattoos the dollar store has to offer. I make sure I permanently have one on. The printed caricature of the Three Headed Dragon my therapist Jean gave me is on my bedroom door (please see the Appendix). The concept is extremely

simple as only brilliant things are and I will try to digest it here as successfully and shortly as I can.

The metaphor is used to address the three aspects of alcohol addiction that an addict needs to understand in order to succeed in sobering up and permanently recovering from his addictionS (not only alcohol!!)

They are: Drinking, Thinking and Feeling. Cutting the first head only and not dealing with your feelings and the way you think, turns you into a so called "dry drunk", a person who is abstinent from alcohol (or other drugs) and very far from being sober. You have to cut all three heads in order to recover. Here. End of story.

It hit me so profoundly because I realized on the spot that in the long periods of my previous 'sobriety' (five years being the longest) I had NOT ONE MINUTE of recovery. I was 100% abstinent from alcohol and totally hammered with co-dependency and guilt and shame. I discovered the level of my emotional immaturity and that Monday morning was no picnic. On a physical level sobriety for me is about accumulation of sober time against time of drinking. And above all: the incredibly liberating firm decision to NEVER EVER have another drink of alcohol. For life.

What did I learn about Bipolar Disorder

We all have our ups and downs, our "off" days and our "on" days, but if you're suffering from bipolar disorder, these peaks and valleys are more severe. The symptoms of bipolar disorder can hurt your job and school performance, damage your relationships, and disrupt your daily life. And although bipolar disorder is treatable, many people don't recognize the warning signs and get the help they need. Since bipolar disorder tends to worsen without treatment, it's important to learn what the symptoms look like. Recognizing the problem is the first step to getting it under control. And that is ALL I wanted: get it under control!!

What is bipolar disorder? Bipolar disorder (also known as manic depression) causes serious shifts in mood, energy, thinking, and behavior—from the highs of mania on one extreme, to the lows of depression on the other. More than just a fleeting good or bad mood, the cycles of bipolar disorder last for days, weeks, or months. And unlike ordinary mood swings, the mood changes of bipolar disorder are so intense that they interfere with your ability to function. During a manic episode, a person might impulsively quit a job, charge up huge amounts on credit cards, or feel rested after sleeping two hours. During a depressive episode, the same person might be too tired to get out of bed and full of self-loathing and hopelessness over being unemployed and in debt. The causes of bipolar disorder aren't completely understood, but it often runs in families. The first manic or depressive episode of bipolar disorder usually occurs in the teenage years or early adulthood. The symptoms can be subtle and confusing, so many people with bipolar disorder are overlooked or misdiagnosed—resulting in unnecessary suffering. But with proper treatment and support, you can lead a rich and fulfilling life.

When we grew up my brother's favorite book was "The Amphibian Man"—a Russian science fiction classic by Aleksander Belyayev, first published in 1928. I ended up reading it 10 million times as well. The book tells the story of a young man named Ichtiandr (literally "Fish Man" in Greek) who as a child received a life-saving transplant—a set of shark gills. The operation was performed by his father, Doctor Salvator, a scientist and a maverick surgeon. The experiment was a success but it limited the young man's ability to interact with the world outside his ocean environment. Similar to other works by Beliaev, the book investigates the possibilities of physical survival under extreme conditions, as well as the moral integrity of scientific experiments. It also touches on socialist ideas of improving living conditions for the world's poor. The book is set in Buenos Aires, Argentina.

Please check out the Wikipedia's entry on Alexander Belyayev. I find his life fascinating.

Every time I go for a swim—in a pool, in a sea, in an ocean, in a lake, I always think of Ichtiandr. I ALWAYS wonder what it would be like to be Ichtiandr. (An exception was the Dead Sea in Israel in August 1997 where you can float without sinking because of the immense salt content . . .)

Another big help was Martha Beck's work on the "Steps to Find Your Life's Path". They are:

Step One: Get Still;
Step Two: Know the Truth;
Step Three: Feel Your Soul's Desires;
Step Four: Trust Your Life to Unfold Perfectly.

Please read Martha Beck's books mentioned in the reference section—she offers invaluable insights!!

Brene Brown's work on shame and guilt resilience presented in her book "I Thought it Was Just Me (but it isn't)" and her DVDs opened my eyes when I came to understand that abstinence from alcohol alone doesn't mean recovery. It was so liberating to grasp that there are nuances of what we perceive as guilt and these are shame, humiliation and embarrassment. It was fabulous to learn that guilt can be actually productive whereas shame can be only destructive. When we apologize and plead "guilty", our crimes and mistakes can bring us forward. If we stick to the shame and keep it a secret without sharing it, it immobilizes us and keeps us prisoners for life. There is a whole "Stage 2 Program" in

ACDC dedicated entirely on building shame and guilt resilience. It is a twelve-week program for two hours weekly and it is another amazing product (much more a "free gift") of the Centre. I will let you know what I have learned in this program upon its completion.

Week after week after my graduation from Stage 1 at ACDC in August time started to fly as I joined the flight of recovery initiated by the Centre. My dishwasher cycle of one hour would pass in a few minutes. I started to starve time. I wanted to fly along. I wanted to be part of the 'yatoto' (Bulgarian for flock). But this time I wanted and needed to do the work myself. I didn't want to be dragged along or carried in someone's arms or be brought to the destination in a bag or a suitcase or a coffin. I wanted to fly on my own, with my own wings but knowing that the wind below them is the wind of the yatoto. That I am not really alone, not really on my own, that we fly together, that we are one strong "yato", which has his destination in sight. A yato which simply KEEPS on flying. But the smart way. With the necessary rest, with the proper nutrition, taking its time to stop and smell the roses and time to meditate. I didn't want to fly against the wind anymore. In the opposite direction. Struggling beyond measure, lonely, hungry, angry, tired. I wanted to migrate with my fellow birds. And this time migration would have a purpose—to take me home. For good. I think that home is not necessarily a place. Home is time. In 51 years I lived in 19 different places in Bulgaria, Germany, Finland and Canada. My last move was this weekend—March 10-11, 2012. My new condo is another fabulous penthouse in the same glorious 'Papillon Place', this time a two bedroom corner unit in order to accommodate Chris and hopefully his girlfriend Yuria. Andy is mostly welcome as always.

I used to be mesmerized by airplanes before. During my Airline experience I have been on endless flights. I liked flying. But now I realized I used to like being FLOWN IN to the destination. I didn't want to work at it. I needed to be teleported. Comfortably—to be fed, served, attended. To have a blanket and a bed (but NB!! not on a transatlantic charter flights please and not in the middle of the last 4 seat-row in front of the lavarories between overweight people who have the flu).

For now almost 20 years I call my family overseas every Sunday at 10 AM sharp (5 PM in Bulgaria). It is a long tradition you can tell. For the first time in my life last Sunday I WAS ABLE to ask my brother to stop talking and to listen to me until I am finished. I never did this before. In the 23 years spent abroad I have paid thousands of dollars on long distance calls with my family in Bulgaria (unforgettable 3 CAD per minute in 1993!!) and I was NEVER able to say something that was important ONLY to me. I would listen to details about what my family had for dinner last night etc. What a flight that is today!!

Planet Papillon

Needless to say, the ad for a 'fully furnished penthouse' was published on Kijiji ten minutes before I visited the website at 5.15 PM on Thursday July 21, 2011 after finding out that I am accepted to the Day Treatment Program starting on Monday July 25, 2011. (Yes, we need full details of time and place.) I was the FIRST caller, the name of the condominium was "Papillon Place" and the landlord's name was Grant. Not John, not Michael, not Simon, not Phillip, it was GRANT!! Let me repeat that: ten minutes, Papillon Place, Grant. Now I REALLY want you to think about it: ten minutes, Papillon Place, Grant. Let's elaborate here for a second or two. It brings together into a prism three points:

1. Timing,
2. Butterflies are free,
3. Granting serenity.

Was I by any chance in need of all three? Someone to grant me freedom? Now? Well...

Today me and Mr. Grant Bigelow are great friends. He took me last to Red Lobster for a Christmas get-together and we laughed over beautiful food that if I become famous with my little booklet, he won't have any problems renting out this property in the future for much higher amount of money—it will become a landmark of Mississauga: "Here lived the famous writer Alma C. and tra-lala-la-laaaaa." Grant's entire family is involved in his successful realty business and I admire their class and wonderful manners. He is also the fastest fixer of refrigerators in the world.

Almost immediately after I moved in into Papillon Place on Tuesday July 26, 2011, I started feeling a funny tingling in my fingers, my brain and my soul at the same time. It was definitely an urge of some sort, but I couldn't figure it out at all. I thought it was a sheer nervousness from being in a new place plus the guilt of leaving Andy, the Cat and the house behind, but the confusing thing was that such "negative" emotions felt actually very good and awfully right . . . . For the first two weeks or so, I had persistent dreams of Gabriel García Márquez' novel "One Hundred Years of Solitude"—my favorite book of all times—which I knew almost by heart in English and in Bulgarian and I kept buying it as a gift for friends (and family, Andy: Christmas 2002—see photo in the appendix, hahaaa), ONLY to be able to dedicate it as: "Aahhh, to you, my dear X, from Alma, terribly envious that you are going to enjoy the greatest privilege of reading this masterpiece for the FIRST time . . . ." And snobbish crap like that. Anyway, the thought of the book and Marquez chased me systematically for the first two weeks in my new nest for some weird reason and honestly, on Friday August 12, 2011—the day I graduated from the Day Treatment intensive care, entering the apartment, it hit me: I figured out what was circling in my brain. I remembered reading long time ago how Marquez wanted to write a book about his grandparents' house since he was eighteen years old but couldn't find the right tone for years. And all of a sudden in 1965, going to Acapulco on a vacation with his family and entering the hotel room, he got literally STRUCK by the idea and that tone!! They had to return home and he wrote for 18 months straight, smoking in his room and letting his family borrow money for food while finishing it and also selling his car to give his wife money for food. Well, c'mon now, I know what you are thinking and no, I am not THAT silly: I am far from implying here that I have anything in common with Marquez (except for chain-smoking) or that "Good Midnight, Insomniacs" is gonna win me the Nobel prize for literature or self-help, but please KNOW that I got the exact same feeling entering my place and taking a deep breath (I mean lighting a cigarette) and breathing in the atmosphere of PH 6: I suddenly KNEW that I will write a book right here and right now, a dream and a plan of mine since grade 1 1967 in Sofia. I just realized that in a very matter-of-fact fashion and it was no big bang, just a big relief and it brought a big smile to my face.

How on earth can you not believe every single word of Marquez' magical realism in his "One Hundred Years of Solitude"?? It surely was real and it definitely felt like magic.

Now you know about that too.

What started as a lifeless ad on a website, turned later into my Planet Papillon. I made sure I populated my planet richly with wonders and great people. A bonus: the dogs were given! I never saw a building with so many dogs—occupants in my life! Today I know them all—by name and owner. My absolute favorite is Christina's Cupcake. Meeting so many dogs here reminded me though of the sad fact that in 33 Harbour Square, a posh condominium where I lived for 14 years between 1993 and 2006, there were no dogs allowed. Not even cats, but we all had cats, and the kids were not allowed to trick or treat for Halloween. Chris was 3 years old when we moved in there and went to the Island Public School from grade 1 till grade 6. He took the glorious ONGIARA ferry boat every morning for 7 years and honestly missed one or two days from school. At that time we still had Romy Schneider—our Siamese cat with the biggest most beautiful blue eyes on earth and the leather chocolate nose. This brings memories indeed, so I could write another 20 pages on Romy alone, but one thing to mention about her is that in Helsinki in 1991 when she was a baby, I took her to the vet because she had horrible heats. In the Cats encyklopedia Siamese cats were proclaimed to be the nymphomaniacs of cats ... Geez, so I took her to the clinic and after the doctor prescribed some hormones for her we left and I brought home the papers. My Finnish was not good at the time and the doctor's English was as poor, so we ended up mixing up the names. The note said that "Alma Botcharova—a Siamese cat with owner Romy Schneider—has a horrible heat and needs medical attention and should be treated with hormones." For years my Finnish neighbors used to greet me in the morning with: "Meow, Alma dear, how is your heat today? Did you get your fix?"

Nevermind, Romy Schneider was the most loved cat in the entire world and Ahi's best buddy for 17 years. She died on August 25, 2007. Nothing is the same ever since. Our new cat—born on May 10, 2009—is as silly as can be.

Back to Planet Papillon and its population. The very first butterfly I met one early morning in the gym was Tiffany—a busy bee, flying around greeting everybody because she is a volunteer in organizing the social events and recreation activities of the residents. Today Tiffany is my best friend in Papillon Place and we exercise together every chance we get. I mostly observe her yoga practice in the mornings, because she is diligent and advanced and I just like to talk to her and discuss life and not so much to stretch in impossible to do postures. But we laugh a lot together, she has the most wonderful smile and a great sense of humor. I joined her on one night for games in the party room and met her many other friends. I am bugging her to convince the Manager of the Recreation Center to buy a table tennis top and put it on one of the two billiard tables so that I can smash her in table tennis since I was a high school champion, but she says that the Manager would NEVER agree to that. I have no way of checking that out. Tiffany came to my first talk at an AA open meeting on October 15, 2011 at the Meadowvale group in Inlake Road and that meant so much to me. She sat in the first row with another very special friend of mine and I felt so proud to have them both sitting there and listening to my story. Tiffany is a great mother and a wonderful wife. She has a little problem with her parking spot underground because she keeps scratching every car her husband buys at the exact same spot. And, although she loves cheesecake, she often says no to my offering her some, because her figure is more important to her than nurturing my obsession with feeding people idiotically. Tiffany is also very cautious regarding material possessions and keeps giving away things non-stop. At the same time, she refuses to accept even the tiniest gift. I love Tiffany dearly and hope she will be my neighbor for a long time. She introduced me to many of our fellow residents and when I head home from work, I feel that I am coming to a place where I know many people whom I am glad to see and they seem glad to see me.

I stopped being afraid of waking up early (anytime between 4 and 5 am) because now I knew that Jackie is already in the gym. Every single day between 5 and 7 AM this Chinese lady would exercise with the determination and devotion of an Olympic champion: 30 minutes treadmill, 15 minutes weights, 15 minutes bike, 10 minutes ball, 10 minutes push-ups, 30 min swim and 10 min sauna. Every single day, no weekends, no holidays excluded. A 63-years—old mother of five and grandmother of fourteen. Jackie, my fitness champion. Actually, as we speak, Jackie's daughter Kim is pregnant in her 9 month and in early January is going to have a baby boy—grandson number 14 for Jackie. I met Kim in the pool a few mornings. Diligent and responsible for her health and her son's health.

My brave next door neighbors Magda and Rafael are two Polish gems. We like the same music, love each other's cuisine, tend to overdo the dancing at our parties (security alert) and laugh a lot together. They are like my niece and nephew—PRECISELY the same age and their biggest importance is that they are here and now. And close. Next door. Such a great feeling to know that they are 6 meters away from me. I understand them completely when they speak in Polish. AA1—my best friend in AA and my sober sister is Polish as well, so I am advancing fast in this crazy language with words containing sometimes 7 consonants without a vowel in between. AA1 is the main character of my SOBER CHAOS sitcom. She is my golden mine.

My favorite Shannelle is a girl from Africa I get a hug from each morning on my way to work. Spiritual, beautiful, energetic, she has an amazing voice and sings in her church's choir. This still remains to be attended but I often hear her singing in the hallway and this is like angel's music to my ears.

There is one more person I would like to mention here who is not a Papillon Place resident and who made such a lasting impression on me: Mrs. Eva Kekis. Eva is an 86 years old lady born in Ukraine whom I met in early September. A close friend of mine asked me to help Eva with her tax return. I needed to translate the forms from German into English because they came from Germany where Eva worked for a few years after the Second World War and was a pension recipient for many years. I did this 32-page translation pro bono and this is something both Eva and my friend claim they will never forget. The more important thing is that I got to meet her. She is the most impressive 86-year-old lady I have ever had a chance to talk to. Always in perfect shape—hair-dressed, elegant, clean, beautiful, simply strong and independent. There is a picture of Eva in my Appendix.

Recently she had another by-pass and recovered successfully thanks to her enormous spiritual (and physical) strength. It is always a pleasure to visit her and chat with her in her impeccably clean house in downtown Toronto where she lives since 1957. This was before I was born. She still bakes her own cookies and is an instant coffee connoisseur. She even allows me to smoke inside her house. She says that she prays for my health every single day. Sometimes when it's slippery and I wear high heels and lose my balance but manage not to fall, I know that this is because Eva asks her God to keep me safe and cracking. She keeps promising to visit me in Mississauga and since we celebrate Easter on the same Sunday maybe this year she will finally let me drive her over here and we might color some eggs together. Or bake some 'kosunatsi" (Bulgarian for Easter bread).

I keep thinking of English Surgeon Sir Frederick Treves (1853-1923) who must have said: "Don't bother about genius. Don't worry about being clever. Trust to hard work, perseverance and determination."

Living On The Hyphen: Curse Or Blessing?

Freud says that you can ALWAYS blame your parents. In order to conquer their own inferiority complex of a small nation, mine locked us up with my brother in a German kindergarten at the age of three. From that period I kept my very firm handshake and numerous stubborn nightmares. As you know by now, my brother became a psychiatrist. At any rate we were brought up bilingual in Bulgarian and German. I've earned my Ph.D. in German Studies and Culture from the University of Toronto, Canada in January 2005. I have my M.A. in Germanistik from Humboldt University Berlin, Germany and my B.A. in German Philology from "Kliment Ohridski" University in Sofia, Bulgaria. In addition to German and English, I am fluent in Russian (all East-Europeans of my generation are) and I have reading knowledge of French (Oh Canada) and Finnish.

I can hardly offer any fresh insights about "living on the hyphen", but I must admit that it has fed me and my son ever since we immigrated to Canada. While still in grad school in 2001, I started my cross-cultural consulting life as an Associate of "Coghill & Beery International", a company for Intercultural Management Consulting based in London, England. We had projects in Canada, England and the USA. I couldn't travel easily during the academic months (SEP—APR), so we did a lot of work online. In any case this wonderful company baptized me by fire and we still work together occasionally. In 2007 after my contract with UofT was up in April and I was facing four summer months with no salary and monstrous student loans repayments, I decided to finally establish my own modest cross-cultural consultancy called—what else—but: "Living on the Hyphen International" (LHI). Through LHI, I want to help international companies and individuals develop cross-cultural competencies and acquire skills to cope with cross-cultural stress for better global competitive advantage and for personal wellbeing and happiness. I believe that the hyphen between our 'home' culture and 'our' target culture (i.e. Bulgarian-Canadian) should not be perceived as a "MINUS" (apart from its diacritical sign), but it can and it should be turned into a major, significant and vital "PLUS"!! Furthermore, I am convinced that in today's world there is not one single person, who is not 'hyphenated' in one form or another. Just look around you, look at your own family and within yourself.

I also realized I need a business partner. It is imperative. I don't think one can succeed on their own. So, LHI is in the making. The idea of such a consultancy has been a great hope through all the years of grad school, part-timing and my imaginary "life after the Ph.D.". There was a vivid sense of initiative associated with LHI in my mind and it constantly increased over the years. LHI is a "sanity-island" ever since it has been started. I actually went so far that I bought the copyright for a live TV talk show with the same title and dreamt of becoming the next Oprah.

Sober Love

This is the shortest chapter in my modest booklet. Since I sobered up THIS TIME!!, I learned only one thing: the opposite of love is not hate, but indifference. Make your own thoughts about it. I am enjoying the liberating effect of this realization every single day and honestly cannot get enough of it. It seems that happiness is a skill after all and being a skill, it can be learnt!! How cool is that? You don't have to be BORN happy (or miserable), you can acquire it as a skill and then practice it every day as much as you want. If you choose not to, you are welcome as well. We only get what we want. "Should" is out of my vocabulary. No more "shoulds" for me, thank you very much. "I want, I would like, I love . . ."—yes, just no more "I should".

As far as sex is concerned, let's just say that since July last year the range in age of the men I have met who are interested in a "closer" relationship with me is 65 years: the oldest man that flirts with me is 83 and the youngest is 28. And everybody in between. Thank you, gentlemen! You are really kind. It will take a long while to recover from my codependency issues, but I am working on them, so don't give up hope. Give me a decade or so.

First we take Manhattan, then we take Berlin!!

Eternal Emails

25 January 2012

My dear Stepping Stones Treasures,

You know, during this first truly sober winter I have sometimes days where I act as if I'm a Nobel prize winner. If I am not booked to go to court, I would get up at noon, have coffee for an hour, go for a swim, then to the sauna, then return home where on a very nice music background I would have something really nice to eat, then a small tiny nap, then more tea, probably a short walk out and back to wait for the boys to come and eat dinner with me. I wouldn't pick up the phone on those days. It's especially nice when it's snowy and horrible outside. The problem is that sometimes such a day can prolong itself into a week, and sometimes into a month, it had happened in the past. Okay, you understand that is a little secret between us. I'm sure Andy and Chris are very suspicious, but hey—that's Canada—innocent until proven guilty!

Good morning my precious SS-Ladies,

I need to report to you on the continuation of my Tuesday night. At Tuesday night's Streetsville AA open meeting I had to LITERALLY ask for my 9 month chip, because the gentleman who was chairing simply skipped the 9-month-recognition by accident (he forgot all about it and started from 6 months). So after he went through 6, 3, 2, 1 month and nobody picked up any of those, a fellow named Andy (pleaseeeee) was the only one who picked a desire chip. After that was done, the chair tried to move on and I started waving from the very back of the room and he said: "Someone is waving at me from way over there.... What do you want, young lady???" And I got up and said:" Uhhh, sorry, Sir, do you mind giving me a 9-month chip because I am afraid you skipped it." The whole room burst into laughter and they were screaming: 'Yes, yes, you forgot it....' Then he asked me loudly about my name and now EVERYBODY knew who I was, asking for my chip. Hahaaaaa ... Great embarrassment and fun at the same time. The culmination was that the two people who picked up a chip that night were "Andy and Alma" (pleaseeeeee Andyyy!!!: my husband's name!!!!!) and we built an "A & A" name combination (Alcoholics Anonymous). Maybe not a miracle, but a magic circumstance for sure. That's my daily report, haaaaaa.

CONCLUSION

When people ask me nowadays what do I do for living, I tell them that I wear a few hats. I have one full time job and a couple of freelance jobs. At 51, I tell them, after graduating from The Addictions and Concurrent Disorders Centre at Credit Valley Hospital in Mississauga I FINALLY got the job of my dreams: I work FULL TIME EVERY SINGLE DAY as a discovering alcoholic and a recovering bipolar patient. I have many work places: ACDC, AA, WFS, SS, DRA, etc. I am occupied 24/7. Among many other things, today I have AA66 who calls me "my sponsor" and "my Mom", I have purpose and I experience joy again. I have some substance and I have a lot of hope. I have my new top gun camera REBEL and I am getting serious about photography. I have my sunrises and please be sure that I will publish some spectacular shots once I finish a course or two at Henry's. I have a lot of reasons to wake up each morning, you see. I get a full Inbox in my email and I am looking forward to respond. I care for others. I am no longer alone and many people tell me they are glad we've met. I am there for my son, and I am not a selfish drunk any longer. I landed on Planet Papillon and I am planning to stay here. I turned the hyphen into a circle. That's one BUSY full time occupation, no? And yes, I remember well: it's really one day at a time. It works for me.

Then I have my freelance jobs: Firstly, I am a freelance court interpreter for the Ministry of the Attorney General of Ontario and let the Bulgarian criminals in Ontario feed me and my family. Sad, but profitable. The stories in the court houses will be published 'post mortum" to avoid trouble. And secondly, I teach German Language, Literature and Culture as a Sessional Lecturer at the German department of the University of Toronto. I stick religiously to this freelance status because it gives me extra time and freedom. I still teach downtown at St. George Campus and need to commute because the beautiful Erindale Campus of UofT lost its program in German Studies a few years ago. That would have been perfect—I live 3 km away from Mississauga Road and Collegeway. Nevermind, the whole 'German' involvement is described in my short story "Frau Doktor Bindestrich" and it is not part of this letter.

In the "Big Book" of AA there are the 'Promises' and I will quote them here:

> "We are going to know a new freedom and a new happiness. We will not regret the past nor wish to shut the door on it. We will comprehend the word serenity and we will know peace. No matter how far down the scale we have gone, we will see how our experience can benefit others. That feeling of uselessness and self-pity will disappear. We will lose interest in selfish things and gain interest in our fellows. Are these extravagant promises? We think not. They are being fulfilled among us—sometimes quickly. Sometimes slowly. They will always materialize if we work for them."

As you may recall, in August 2011 my goal became to achieve a better ending of my life instead of a brand new beginning. (Menopause helped a lot in defining this goal. The hormonal turmoil wouldn't let me choose my teen age over life after 50. THE BEST IS TRULY YET TO COME!) Anyways, let the wonderful topic of menopause not make me lose my male readers just before the end of my letter to you. My men AA fellows suffer enough from my hot flashes and my insomnia. So here is the ultimate conclusion:

I seem to have started discovering the butterfly in me. May you start discovering yours today. Fly to your Pink Cloud and embrace it. Or swim to it. Whatever works for you. (And what a great movie that is by Woody Allen "Whatever works"—check it out.) In any case: any action is better than inaction. Any action on your part will take you to your Pink Cloud. What a feeling that is!!

Once I started my butterflying journey towards my now quite unmodest goal "the BEST POSSIBLE ending of my life", something took me by surprise. I must admit that working on the ending turns out to be a daily, constant, empowering and energetic beginning of some sort. One rebirth after another. Funny. I guess we have a word for re-birth but not for re-death after all. As Scarlett O'Hara puts it in "Gone with the winds": "Ater all, tomorrow ia another day." My discovery reads: "After all, TODAY is another day."

Thank you for reading my letter. Please write back. What are you up to today? Let me know.

I am off to Youtube to listen to Barbra Streisand's song "Memory" again and then check out the Dollarama for Valentine's Day. For me discount stores have more than enough glitter and pink items. It doesn't cost you a fortune to celebrate any holiday during the year and to make someone smile.

Yours warmly,
Alma

P.S. Signing my letter to you made me realize that when I say "I am Alma" lately, I feel like I know who I am and what I talk about starts to make more sense to me. How weird is that? If I go back to my brother's motto-quote at the beginning of this letter, yes: I must be one of the people "overdoing being insane". But you know what: it's much better than under-doing it or NOT doing it at all. Trust me on that one. All it takes is for us to HONESTLY figure out where we stand, then decide what is right and stick to it. Make a plan and stay the course.

Romain Rolland said: "A hero is a man who does what he can." Precisely.

RECOMMENDATIONS and REFERENCES

I created (let someone create, I mean) a website with the full list of resources, recommendations and references. Please visit www.aaa.com.

Here are some immediate ideas. And they are NOT in alphabetical order. They are listed rather according to their importance to me or even the order I have read them since I started my recovery in July 2011.

Spirituality and Wellbeing:

The beginning of my spiritual journey brought me back to the work of hopefully not forgotten Bulgarian Master Beinsa Duno (Peter Deunov). I was familiar with his writings as early as 1980ies. In the university in Sofia he was considered the most prominent Bulgarian philosopher and spiritual teacher. It's amazing what a totally new resonance I discovered reading his books again last summer over thirty years later and from a new point of view (search). As a brand new member of AA I remember being "kindly pushed" by the requirement of finding my Higher Power "soon please" and I clearly recall constantly thinking: "Where the heck are you hiding, my Dear?" So I kept rereading the Big Book of AA, searching and searching. Then one evening—August 27, 2011 to be precise as always, hmmmm—when I was packing my "most important" books from the house in order to bring them to my new condo, I saw Peter Dunov's books in Bulgarian and grabbed them all. I read all night and had a big smile: Welcome Buddy! I got you!

Just read the following excerpt please:

"People want to attribute a certain form to God, but I ask the question what form can you attribute to Light? Light itself creates forms. How does it create forms? As soon as it encounters an obstacle, it already creates a certain form. Make the environment of your thoughts rarer or denser and they will immediately experience some refraction." (Youth Class, year I, lecture 5, *Old and New Lives*, (29 March 1922)

In the following days I was stunned to see how popular my Master was in North America—the Wikipedia entry stroke me as so objective and made me proud to be Bulgarian. I firmly believe that Peter Deunov's teachings are the foundation of the work by numerous North-American thinkers and new-age teachers such as Joseph Murphy, author of "The Power of Your Subconscious Mind" and Rhonda Byrne, author of "The Secret" to name just a couple. The similarity in the train of thought is just stunning. You can find a lot of information online on Peter Deunov. Please give it a search, it's more than gainful.

What I figured out is that there is such a big difference between religion and spirituality! The Latin "religio" means as much as "to tie, to bond", whereas "spiritus" means among other things "to breathe" in the sense of "the act of being filled with air". So in the case of 'religion', man enters a contract with his God. This is a very personal deal. If man is 'spiritual' on the other hand, he/ she learns how to share the air with everybody else on earth.

Burt Goldman: **THE AMERICAN MONK.**

MUSIC:

British chart-toppers Mika and Adele

TV:

The Office
The Daily Show

The Colbert Report
Conan
All Comedy channels
Blue Collar Radio

BOOKS:

Azade Seyhan: "Writing Outside the Nation"
"The Big Book of Alcoholics Anonymous"
Frederic Flach: "The Secret Strength of Depression"
Charlotte Davis Kasl: "Many Roads, One Journey: Moving Beyond the 12 Steps"
—; "Yes You Can: Healing from Trauma and Addiction with Love, Strength, and Power"
Caroline Knapp: "Drinking, A Love Story"
Joseph Murphy: 'The Power of Your Subconscious Mind" Rhonda Byrne: "The Secret"
Colleen E. Carney & Rachel Manber: "Quiet Your Mind and Get to Sleep"
Bob Stahl & Elisha Goldstein: "A Mindfulness-Based Stress Reduction Workbook"
Dennis Greenberger and Christine A. Padesky: "Mind Over Mood: Change How You Feel by Changing the Way You Think"
Gretchen Rubin: "The Happiness Project"
Robin Shrama: "The Secret Letters of the Monk who sold his Ferrari"
Jon Kabat-Zinn: "Wherever You Go There You Are"
Jeannette Walls: "The Glass Castle"
John Izzo: "Stepping Up: How Taking Responsibility Changes Everything"
Rick Warren: "Purpose Driven: What on Earth Am I Here for?"
Tyrese Gibson: "How to Get Out of Your Own Way"
Lish Osteen Comes: "You Are Made for More"

Mark Nepo: "The Book of Awakening" (Having the Life you want by being Present to the Life You Have)
Mitch Albom: "Have a Little Faith"
—— "Tuesdays with Morrie"

Norman Vincent Peale: "The Power of Positive Thinking"
—"The Amazing results of Positive Thinking"
Neil Pasricha: "The Book of Awesome"
Don Miguel Ruiz: "The Four Arguments"
Sheeba Varghese: "Sheeba's Secret: A Formula for More Success Through Greater Self-Awareness"
Sigued: "Remember, There is Always more"
Paul T. Mason & Randi Kreger: "Stop Walking on Eggshells"
David J. Schwartz: "The Magic of Thinking Big"
Paul Wiekes: "The Art of Confession; Renewing Yourself Through the Practice of Honesty"
Susan Jeffers: "Feel the Fear and Do IT Anyway; Dynamic Techniques for turning fear, indecision, and anger into power, action and love"
Derek Liu: "The Tao of Joy Every Day: 365 Days of Tao Living"
Claire Dederer: "Poser: My Life in Twenty-Three Yoga Poses"
Rick Hanson: "Just One Thing: Developing a Buddha Brain One Simple Practice at a Time"
Melody Beattie: "Make Miracles in Forty Days: Thinking What You Have Into What You Want"
Brene Brown: "I Thought It Was Just Me (but it isn't)"
Martha Beck: "Finding Your Own North Star"
—"Find Your Way in a Wild New World: Reclaim Your True Nature to Create the Life You Want"
Lisa Bloom: "Think: Straight talk for Women to Stay Smart in a Dumbed-Down World"
Martin E. P. Seligman: "Authentic Happiness"
—"A Visionary New Understanding of Happiness and Well-being"

Joel Osteen: "Everyday a Friday: How to be happier 7 days a Week"

Jack Canfield: "The Success Principles: How to Get From Where You Are to Where You Want to Be"

Byron Katie: "Loving What Is: Four Questions that Can Change Your Life"

Debbie Macomber: "One Word Can Make All the Difference: One Perfect Word"

Lee Lipsenthal: "Enjoy Every Living SaR. Covey: "ndwich Each Day as if it Were Your Last"

Karen Armstrong: "Twelve Steps to a Compassionate Life"

Louise Hay: "Heal Your Life"

Sophy Burnham: "The Art of Intuition: Cultivating Your Inner Wisdom"

Stephen R. Covey: "The 7 Habits of Highly Effective People"

Rob Bell: "Love Wins"

Lori Deschene: "Tiny Buddha: Simple Wisdom for Life's Hard Questions"

PHOTO ALBUMS

LA PAPILLON PLACE

LINKS:

http://www.kodakgallery.ca/ShareLanding.action?c=8ea2vss9.hl6188vd&x=0&y=b7qbd5&localeid=en_CA

http://family.webshots.com/album/582304666yLbhwh

http://family.webshots.com/album/582291507oKfmIE

CPSIA information can be obtained at www.ICGtesting.com
Printed in the USA
LVOW041110030512

279909LV00003B/4/P

9 781469 778334